This book belongs to:

Date _______________ Start time _________ End time _________

Course Name	
Weather	Temp
Handicap	Par
Tees	Yardage
Players	

Front 9

Holes	Par	Drive	Fairway	Putts	Hazard	Yardage	Strokes
1							
2							
3							
4							
5							
6							
7							
8							
9							
Total							

Back 9

Holes	Par	Drive	Fairway	Putts	Hazard	Yardage	Strokes
10							
11							
12							
13							
14							
15							
16							
17							
18							
Total							
Grand Total							

Albatross	Eagles	Birdies	Pars	Bogeys	Doubles	Triples

Notes

Date _________________ Start time _________ End time _________

Course Name	
Weather	Temp
Handicap	Par
Tees	Yardage
Players	

Front 9							
Holes	Par	Drive	Fairway	Putts	Hazard	Yardage	Strokes
1							
2							
3							
4							
5							
6							
7							
8							
9							
Total							
Back 9							
10							
11							
12							
13							
14							
15							
16							
17							
18							
Total							
Grand Total							

	Albatross	Eagles	Birdies	Pars	Bogeys	Doubles	Triples

Notes

Date _______________ Start time _________ End time _________

Course Name

Weather   Temp

Handicap   Par

Tees   Yardage

Players

Front 9							
Holes	Par	Drive	Fairway	Putts	Hazard	Yardage	Strokes
1							
2							
3							
4							
5							
6							
7							
8							
9							
Total							
Back 9							
10							
11							
12							
13							
14							
15							
16							
17							
18							
Total							
Grand Total							

Albatross	Eagles	Birdies	Pars	Bogeys	Doubles	Triples

Notes

Date _______________ Start time _________ End time _________

Course Name

Weather ________________________ Temp

Handicap ________________________ Par

Tees ________________________ Yardage

Players

Front 9

Holes	Par	Drive	Fairway	Putts	Hazard	Yardage	Strokes
1							
2							
3							
4							
5							
6							
7							
8							
9							
Total							

Back 9

Holes	Par	Drive	Fairway	Putts	Hazard	Yardage	Strokes
10							
11							
12							
13							
14							
15							
16							
17							
18							
Total							
Grand Total							

Albatross	Eagles	Birdies	Pars	Bogeys	Doubles	Triples

Notes

Course Name

Weather   Temp

Handicap   Par

Tees   Yardage

Players

Front 9							
Holes	Par	Drive	Fairway	Putts	Hazard	Yardage	Strokes
1							
2							
3							
4							
5							
6							
7							
8							
9							
Total							
Back 9							
10							
11							
12							
13							
14							
15							
16							
17							
18							
Total							
Grand Total							

Albatross	Eagles	Birdies	Pars	Bogeys	Doubles	Triples

Notes

Date ________________ Start time _________ End time _________

Course Name	
Weather	Temp
Handicap	Par
Tees	Yardage
Players	

Front 9

Holes	Par	Drive	Fairway	Putts	Hazard	Yardage	Strokes
1							
2							
3							
4							
5							
6							
7							
8							
9							
Total							

Back 9

10							
11							
12							
13							
14							
15							
16							
17							
18							
Total							
Grand Total							

Albatross	Eagles	Birdies	Pars	Bogeys	Doubles	Triples

Notes

Date _______________ Start time _________ End time _________

Course Name	
Weather	Temp
Handicap	Par
Tees	Yardage
Players	

Front 9

Holes	Par	Drive	Fairway	Putts	Hazard	Yardage	Strokes
1							
2							
3							
4							
5							
6							
7							
8							
9							
Total							

Back 9

Holes	Par	Drive	Fairway	Putts	Hazard	Yardage	Strokes
10							
11							
12							
13							
14							
15							
16							
17							
18							
Total							
Grand Total							

Albatross	Eagles	Birdies	Pars	Bogeys	Doubles	Triples

Notes

Date _________________ Start time _________ End time _________

Course Name		
Weather	Temp	
Handicap	Par	
Tees	Yardage	
Players		

Front 9

Holes	Par	Drive	Fairway	Putts	Hazard	Yardage	Strokes
1							
2							
3							
4							
5							
6							
7							
8							
9							
Total							

Back 9

Holes	Par	Drive	Fairway	Putts	Hazard	Yardage	Strokes
10							
11							
12							
13							
14							
15							
16							
17							
18							
Total							
Grand Total							

	Albatross	Eagles	Birdies	Pars	Bogeys	Doubles	Triples

Notes

Date _________________ Start time _________ End time _________

Course Name ______________________________

Weather ____________________ Temp ________________

Handicap __________________ Par _________________

Tees ______________________ Yardage _____________

Players ___________________________________

<table>
<tr><td colspan="8" align="center">Front 9</td></tr>
<tr><td>Holes</td><td>Par</td><td>Drive</td><td>Fairway</td><td>Putts</td><td>Hazard</td><td>Yardage</td><td>Strokes</td></tr>
<tr><td>1</td><td></td><td></td><td></td><td></td><td></td><td></td><td></td></tr>
<tr><td>2</td><td></td><td></td><td></td><td></td><td></td><td></td><td></td></tr>
<tr><td>3</td><td></td><td></td><td></td><td></td><td></td><td></td><td></td></tr>
<tr><td>4</td><td></td><td></td><td></td><td></td><td></td><td></td><td></td></tr>
<tr><td>5</td><td></td><td></td><td></td><td></td><td></td><td></td><td></td></tr>
<tr><td>6</td><td></td><td></td><td></td><td></td><td></td><td></td><td></td></tr>
<tr><td>7</td><td></td><td></td><td></td><td></td><td></td><td></td><td></td></tr>
<tr><td>8</td><td></td><td></td><td></td><td></td><td></td><td></td><td></td></tr>
<tr><td>9</td><td></td><td></td><td></td><td></td><td></td><td></td><td></td></tr>
<tr><td>Total</td><td></td><td></td><td></td><td></td><td></td><td></td><td></td></tr>
<tr><td colspan="8" align="center">Back 9</td></tr>
<tr><td>10</td><td></td><td></td><td></td><td></td><td></td><td></td><td></td></tr>
<tr><td>11</td><td></td><td></td><td></td><td></td><td></td><td></td><td></td></tr>
<tr><td>12</td><td></td><td></td><td></td><td></td><td></td><td></td><td></td></tr>
<tr><td>13</td><td></td><td></td><td></td><td></td><td></td><td></td><td></td></tr>
<tr><td>14</td><td></td><td></td><td></td><td></td><td></td><td></td><td></td></tr>
<tr><td>15</td><td></td><td></td><td></td><td></td><td></td><td></td><td></td></tr>
<tr><td>16</td><td></td><td></td><td></td><td></td><td></td><td></td><td></td></tr>
<tr><td>17</td><td></td><td></td><td></td><td></td><td></td><td></td><td></td></tr>
<tr><td>18</td><td></td><td></td><td></td><td></td><td></td><td></td><td></td></tr>
<tr><td>Total</td><td></td><td></td><td></td><td></td><td></td><td></td><td></td></tr>
<tr><td>Grand Total</td><td></td><td></td><td></td><td></td><td></td><td></td><td></td></tr>
</table>

Albatross	Eagles	Birdies	Pars	Bogeys	Doubles	Triples

Notes

Date _______________ Start time _________ End time _______

Course Name	
Weather	Temp
Handicap	Par
Tees	Yardage
Players	

Front 9

Holes	Par	Drive	Fairway	Putts	Hazard	Yardage	Strokes
1							
2							
3							
4							
5							
6							
7							
8							
9							
Total							

Back 9

Holes	Par	Drive	Fairway	Putts	Hazard	Yardage	Strokes
10							
11							
12							
13							
14							
15							
16							
17							
18							
Total							
Grand Total							

Albatross	Eagles	Birdies	Pars	Bogeys	Doubles	Triples

Notes

Date _________________ Start time _________ End time _________

Course Name	
Weather	Temp
Handicap	Par
Tees	Yardage
Players	

Front 9							
Holes	Par	Drive	Fairway	Putts	Hazard	Yardage	Strokes
1							
2							
3							
4							
5							
6							
7							
8							
9							
Total							

Back 9							
10							
11							
12							
13							
14							
15							
16							
17							
18							
Total							
Grand Total							

Albatross	Eagles	Birdies	Pars	Bogeys	Doubles	Triples

Notes

Date _______________ Start time _________ End time _________

Course Name	
Weather	Temp
Handicap	Par
Tees	Yardage
Players	

Front 9

Holes	Par	Drive	Fairway	Putts	Hazard	Yardage	Strokes
1							
2							
3							
4							
5							
6							
7							
8							
9							
Total							

Back 9

Holes	Par	Drive	Fairway	Putts	Hazard	Yardage	Strokes
10							
11							
12							
13							
14							
15							
16							
17							
18							
Total							
Grand Total							

Albatross	Eagles	Birdies	Pars	Bogeys	Doubles	Triples

Notes

Date _______________ Start time _________ End time _________

Course Name

Weather	Temp
Handicap	Par
Tees	Yardage
Players	

Front 9

Holes	Par	Drive	Fairway	Putts	Hazard	Yardage	Strokes
1							
2							
3							
4							
5							
6							
7							
8							
9							
Total							

Back 9

Holes	Par	Drive	Fairway	Putts	Hazard	Yardage	Strokes
10							
11							
12							
13							
14							
15							
16							
17							
18							
Total							
Grand Total							

Albatross	Eagles	Birdies	Pars	Bogeys	Doubles	Triples

Notes

Date _______________ Start time _________ End time _________

Course Name	
Weather	Temp
Handicap	Par
Tees	Yardage
Players	

Front 9							
Holes	Par	Drive	Fairway	Putts	Hazard	Yardage	Strokes
1							
2							
3							
4							
5							
6							
7							
8							
9							
Total							
Back 9							
10							
11							
12							
13							
14							
15							
16							
17							
18							
Total							
Grand Total							

	Albatross	Eagles	Birdies	Pars	Bogeys	Doubles	Triples

Notes

Date _________________ Start time _________ End time _________

Course Name	
Weather	Temp
Handicap	Par
Tees	Yardage
Players	

Front 9

Holes	Par	Drive	Fairway	Putts	Hazard	Yardage	Strokes
1							
2							
3							
4							
5							
6							
7							
8							
9							
Total							

Back 9

Holes	Par	Drive	Fairway	Putts	Hazard	Yardage	Strokes
10							
11							
12							
13							
14							
15							
16							
17							
18							
Total							
Grand Total							

Albatross	Eagles	Birdies	Pars	Bogeys	Doubles	Triples

Notes

Date _______________ Start time _________ End time _________

Course Name	
Weather	Temp
Handicap	Par
Tees	Yardage
Players	

Front 9

Holes	Par	Drive	Fairway	Putts	Hazard	Yardage	Strokes
1							
2							
3							
4							
5							
6							
7							
8							
9							
Total							

Back 9

Holes	Par	Drive	Fairway	Putts	Hazard	Yardage	Strokes
10							
11							
12							
13							
14							
15							
16							
17							
18							
Total							
Grand Total							

	Albatross	Eagles	Birdies	Pars	Bogeys	Doubles	Triples

Notes

Date _________________ Start time _________ End time _________

Course Name	
Weather	Temp
Handicap	Par
Tees	Yardage
Players	

Front 9

Holes	Par	Drive	Fairway	Putts	Hazard	Yardage	Strokes
1							
2							
3							
4							
5							
6							
7							
8							
9							
Total							

Back 9

Holes	Par	Drive	Fairway	Putts	Hazard	Yardage	Strokes
10							
11							
12							
13							
14							
15							
16							
17							
18							
Total							
Grand Total							

Albatross	Eagles	Birdies	Pars	Bogeys	Doubles	Triples

Notes

Date _________________ Start time _________ End time _________

Course Name	
Weather	Temp
Handicap	Par
Tees	Yardage
Players	

Front 9

Holes	Par	Drive	Fairway	Putts	Hazard	Yardage	Strokes
1							
2							
3							
4							
5							
6							
7							
8							
9							
Total							

Back 9

Holes	Par	Drive	Fairway	Putts	Hazard	Yardage	Strokes
10							
11							
12							
13							
14							
15							
16							
17							
18							
Total							
Grand Total							

Albatross	Eagles	Birdies	Pars	Bogeys	Doubles	Triples

Notes

Date _______________ Start time _________ End time _______

Course Name	
Weather	Temp
Handicap	Par
Tees	Yardage
Players	

Front 9

Holes	Par	Drive	Fairway	Putts	Hazard	Yardage	Strokes
1							
2							
3							
4							
5							
6							
7							
8							
9							
Total							

Back 9

Holes	Par	Drive	Fairway	Putts	Hazard	Yardage	Strokes
10							
11							
12							
13							
14							
15							
16							
17							
18							
Total							
Grand Total							

Albatross	Eagles	Birdies	Pars	Bogeys	Doubles	Triples

Notes

Date _________________ Start time _________ End time _________

Course Name

Weather   Temp

Handicap   Par

Tees   Yardage

Players

Front 9

Holes	Par	Drive	Fairway	Putts	Hazard	Yardage	Strokes
1							
2							
3							
4							
5							
6							
7							
8							
9							
Total							

Back 9

Holes	Par	Drive	Fairway	Putts	Hazard	Yardage	Strokes
10							
11							
12							
13							
14							
15							
16							
17							
18							
Total							
Grand Total							

Albatross	Eagles	Birdies	Pars	Bogeys	Doubles	Triples

Notes

Date _________________ Start time _________ End time _________

Course Name	
Weather	Temp
Handicap	Par
Tees	Yardage
Players	

Front 9							
Holes	Par	Drive	Fairway	Putts	Hazard	Yardage	Strokes
1							
2							
3							
4							
5							
6							
7							
8							
9							
Total							

Back 9							
10							
11							
12							
13							
14							
15							
16							
17							
18							
Total							
Grand Total							

Albatross	Eagles	Birdies	Pars	Bogeys	Doubles	Triples

Notes

Date _________________ Start time __________ End time __________

Course Name	
Weather		Temp	
Handicap		Par	
Tees		Yardage	
Players	

Front 9

Holes	Par	Drive	Fairway	Putts	Hazard	Yardage	Strokes
1							
2							
3							
4							
5							
6							
7							
8							
9							
Total							

Back 9

Holes	Par	Drive	Fairway	Putts	Hazard	Yardage	Strokes
10							
11							
12							
13							
14							
15							
16							
17							
18							
Total							
Grand Total							

Albatross	Eagles	Birdies	Pars	Bogeys	Doubles	Triples

Notes

Date _________________ Start time _________ End time _________

Course Name

Weather   Temp

Handicap   Par

Tees   Yardage

Players

Front 9

Holes	Par	Drive	Fairway	Putts	Hazard	Yardage	Strokes
1							
2							
3							
4							
5							
6							
7							
8							
9							
Total							

Back 9

Holes	Par	Drive	Fairway	Putts	Hazard	Yardage	Strokes
10							
11							
12							
13							
14							
15							
16							
17							
18							
Total							
Grand Total							

Albatross	Eagles	Birdies	Pars	Bogeys	Doubles	Triples

Notes

Date ________________ Start time _________ End time _________

Course Name

Weather   Temp

Handicap   Par

Tees   Yardage

Players

Front 9							
Holes	Par	Drive	Fairway	Putts	Hazard	Yardage	Strokes
1							
2							
3							
4							
5							
6							
7							
8							
9							
Total							

Back 9							
10							
11							
12							
13							
14							
15							
16							
17							
18							
Total							
Grand Total							

Albatross	Eagles	Birdies	Pars	Bogeys	Doubles	Triples

Notes

Date _______________ Start time _________ End time _________

Course Name

Weather   Temp

Handicap   Par

Tees   Yardage

Players

Front 9

Holes	Par	Drive	Fairway	Putts	Hazard	Yardage	Strokes
1							
2							
3							
4							
5							
6							
7							
8							
9							
Total							

Back 9

Holes	Par	Drive	Fairway	Putts	Hazard	Yardage	Strokes
10							
11							
12							
13							
14							
15							
16							
17							
18							
Total							
Grand Total							

Albatross	Eagles	Birdies	Pars	Bogeys	Doubles	Triples

Notes

Date _______________ Start time _________ End time _______

Course Name	
Weather	Temp
Handicap	Par
Tees	Yardage
Players	

Front 9

Holes	Par	Drive	Fairway	Putts	Hazard	Yardage	Strokes
1							
2							
3							
4							
5							
6							
7							
8							
9							
Total							

Back 9

Holes	Par	Drive	Fairway	Putts	Hazard	Yardage	Strokes
10							
11							
12							
13							
14							
15							
16							
17							
18							
Total							
Grand Total							

Albatross	Eagles	Birdies	Pars	Bogeys	Doubles	Triples

Notes

Date _________________ Start time _________ End time _________

Course Name

Weather   Temp

Handicap   Par

Tees   Yardage

Players

Front 9							
Holes	Par	Drive	Fairway	Putts	Hazard	Yardage	Strokes
1							
2							
3							
4							
5							
6							
7							
8							
9							
Total							
Back 9							
10							
11							
12							
13							
14							
15							
16							
17							
18							
Total							
Grand Total							

Albatross	Eagles	Birdies	Pars	Bogeys	Doubles	Triples

Notes

Date _______________ Start time _________ End time _________

Course Name	
Weather	Temp
Handicap	Par
Tees	Yardage
Players	

Front 9

Holes	Par	Drive	Fairway	Putts	Hazard	Yardage	Strokes
1							
2							
3							
4							
5							
6							
7							
8							
9							
Total							

Back 9

10							
11							
12							
13							
14							
15							
16							
17							
18							
Total							
Grand Total							

Albatross	Eagles	Birdies	Pars	Bogeys	Doubles	Triples

Notes

Date _______________ Start time _________ End time _________

Course Name

Weather   Temp

Handicap   Par

Tees   Yardage

Players

Front 9							
Holes	Par	Drive	Fairway	Putts	Hazard	Yardage	Strokes
1							
2							
3							
4							
5							
6							
7							
8							
9							
Total							
Back 9							
10							
11							
12							
13							
14							
15							
16							
17							
18							
Total							
Grand Total							

Albatross	Eagles	Birdies	Pars	Bogeys	Doubles	Triples

Notes

Date _______________ Start time _________ End time _________

Course Name	
Weather	Temp
Handicap	Par
Tees	Yardage
Players	

Front 9

Holes	Par	Drive	Fairway	Putts	Hazard	Yardage	Strokes
1							
2							
3							
4							
5							
6							
7							
8							
9							
Total							

Back 9

	Par	Drive	Fairway	Putts	Hazard	Yardage	Strokes
10							
11							
12							
13							
14							
15							
16							
17							
18							
Total							
Grand Total							

Albatross	Eagles	Birdies	Pars	Bogeys	Doubles	Triples

Notes

Date _________________ Start time _________ End time _______

Course Name	
Weather	Temp
Handicap	Par
Tees	Yardage
Players	

Front 9

Holes	Par	Drive	Fairway	Putts	Hazard	Yardage	Strokes
1							
2							
3							
4							
5							
6							
7							
8							
9							
Total							

Back 9

Holes	Par	Drive	Fairway	Putts	Hazard	Yardage	Strokes
10							
11							
12							
13							
14							
15							
16							
17							
18							
Total							
Grand Total							

	Albatross	Eagles	Birdies	Pars	Bogeys	Doubles	Triples

Notes

Date _________________ Start time _________ End time _________

Course Name

Weather   Temp

Handicap   Par

Tees   Yardage

Players

Front 9

Holes	Par	Drive	Fairway	Putts	Hazard	Yardage	Strokes
1							
2							
3							
4							
5							
6							
7							
8							
9							
Total							

Back 9

Holes	Par	Drive	Fairway	Putts	Hazard	Yardage	Strokes
10							
11							
12							
13							
14							
15							
16							
17							
18							
Total							
Grand Total							

Albatross	Eagles	Birdies	Pars	Bogeys	Doubles	Triples

Notes

Date _______________ Start time _________ End time _________

Course Name

Weather   Temp

Handicap   Par

Tees   Yardage

Players

Front 9

Holes	Par	Drive	Fairway	Putts	Hazard	Yardage	Strokes
1							
2							
3							
4							
5							
6							
7							
8							
9							
Total							

Back 9

Holes	Par	Drive	Fairway	Putts	Hazard	Yardage	Strokes
10							
11							
12							
13							
14							
15							
16							
17							
18							
Total							
Grand Total							

Albatross	Eagles	Birdies	Pars	Bogeys	Doubles	Triples

Notes

Date _______________ Start time _________ End time _________

Course Name	
Weather	Temp
Handicap	Par
Tees	Yardage
Players	

Front 9

Holes	Par	Drive	Fairway	Putts	Hazard	Yardage	Strokes
1							
2							
3							
4							
5							
6							
7							
8							
9							
Total							

Back 9

10							
11							
12							
13							
14							
15							
16							
17							
18							
Total							
Grand Total							

Albatross	Eagles	Birdies	Pars	Bogeys	Doubles	Triples

Notes

Date _______________ Start time _________ End time _________

Course Name	
Weather	Temp
Handicap	Par
Tees	Yardage
Players	

Front 9

Holes	Par	Drive	Fairway	Putts	Hazard	Yardage	Strokes
1							
2							
3							
4							
5							
6							
7							
8							
9							
Total							

Back 9

Holes	Par	Drive	Fairway	Putts	Hazard	Yardage	Strokes
10							
11							
12							
13							
14							
15							
16							
17							
18							
Total							
Grand Total							

Albatross	Eagles	Birdies	Pars	Bogeys	Doubles	Triples

Notes

Date _________________ Start time _________ End time _________

Course Name

Weather   Temp

Handicap   Par

Tees   Yardage

Players

Front 9

Holes	Par	Drive	Fairway	Putts	Hazard	Yardage	Strokes
1							
2							
3							
4							
5							
6							
7							
8							
9							
Total							

Back 9

10							
11							
12							
13							
14							
15							
16							
17							
18							
Total							
Grand Total							

Albatross	Eagles	Birdies	Pars	Bogeys	Doubles	Triples

Notes

Date _________________ Start time _________ End time _________

Course Name	
Weather	Temp
Handicap	Par
Tees	Yardage
Players	

Front 9

Holes	Par	Drive	Fairway	Putts	Hazard	Yardage	Strokes
1							
2							
3							
4							
5							
6							
7							
8							
9							
Total							

Back 9

Holes	Par	Drive	Fairway	Putts	Hazard	Yardage	Strokes
10							
11							
12							
13							
14							
15							
16							
17							
18							
Total							
Grand Total							

Albatross	Eagles	Birdies	Pars	Bogeys	Doubles	Triples

Notes

Date _________________ Start time _________ End time _________

Course Name	
Weather	Temp
Handicap	Par
Tees	Yardage
Players	

Front 9

Holes	Par	Drive	Fairway	Putts	Hazard	Yardage	Strokes
1							
2							
3							
4							
5							
6							
7							
8							
9							
Total							

Back 9

Holes	Par	Drive	Fairway	Putts	Hazard	Yardage	Strokes
10							
11							
12							
13							
14							
15							
16							
17							
18							
Total							
Grand Total							

Albatross	Eagles	Birdies	Pars	Bogeys	Doubles	Triples

Notes

Date _________________ Start time _________ End time _________

Course Name	
Weather	Temp
Handicap	Par
Tees	Yardage
Players	

Front 9							
Holes	Par	Drive	Fairway	Putts	Hazard	Yardage	Strokes
1							
2							
3							
4							
5							
6							
7							
8							
9							
Total							
Back 9							
10							
11							
12							
13							
14							
15							
16							
17							
18							
Total							
Grand Total							

Albatross	Eagles	Birdies	Pars	Bogeys	Doubles	Triples

Notes

Date _________________ Start time _________ End time _________

Course Name	
Weather	Temp
Handicap	Par
Tees	Yardage
Players	

Front 9

Holes	Par	Drive	Fairway	Putts	Hazard	Yardage	Strokes
1							
2							
3							
4							
5							
6							
7							
8							
9							
Total							

Back 9

Holes	Par	Drive	Fairway	Putts	Hazard	Yardage	Strokes
10							
11							
12							
13							
14							
15							
16							
17							
18							
Total							
Grand Total							

Albatross	Eagles	Birdies	Pars	Bogeys	Doubles	Triples

Notes

Date _________________ Start time _________ End time _________

Course Name	
Weather	Temp
Handicap	Par
Tees	Yardage
Players	

Front 9

Holes	Par	Drive	Fairway	Putts	Hazard	Yardage	Strokes
1							
2							
3							
4							
5							
6							
7							
8							
9							
Total							

Back 9

Holes	Par	Drive	Fairway	Putts	Hazard	Yardage	Strokes
10							
11							
12							
13							
14							
15							
16							
17							
18							
Total							
Grand Total							

Albatross	Eagles	Birdies	Pars	Bogeys	Doubles	Triples

Notes

Date ________________ Start time _________ End time _________

Course Name	
Weather	Temp
Handicap	Par
Tees	Yardage
Players	

Front 9

Holes	Par	Drive	Fairway	Putts	Hazard	Yardage	Strokes
1							
2							
3							
4							
5							
6							
7							
8							
9							
Total							

Back 9

Holes	Par	Drive	Fairway	Putts	Hazard	Yardage	Strokes
10							
11							
12							
13							
14							
15							
16							
17							
18							
Total							
Grand Total							

Albatross	Eagles	Birdies	Pars	Bogeys	Doubles	Triples

Notes

Date _________________ Start time _________ End time _________

Course Name

Weather   Temp

Handicap   Par

Tees   Yardage

Players

Front 9

Holes	Par	Drive	Fairway	Putts	Hazard	Yardage	Strokes
1							
2							
3							
4							
5							
6							
7							
8							
9							
Total							

Back 9

	Par	Drive	Fairway	Putts	Hazard	Yardage	Strokes
10							
11							
12							
13							
14							
15							
16							
17							
18							
Total							
Grand Total							

Albatross	Eagles	Birdies	Pars	Bogeys	Doubles	Triples

Notes

Date _______________ Start time _________ End time _________

Course Name

Weather   Temp

Handicap   Par

Tees   Yardage

Players

Front 9							
Holes	Par	Drive	Fairway	Putts	Hazard	Yardage	Strokes
1							
2							
3							
4							
5							
6							
7							
8							
9							
Total							
Back 9							
10							
11							
12							
13							
14							
15							
16							
17							
18							
Total							
Grand Total							

Albatross	Eagles	Birdies	Pars	Bogeys	Doubles	Triples

Notes

Date _________________ Start time _________ End time _________

Course Name	
Weather	Temp
Handicap	Par
Tees	Yardage
Players	

Front 9

Holes	Par	Drive	Fairway	Putts	Hazard	Yardage	Strokes
1							
2							
3							
4							
5							
6							
7							
8							
9							
Total							

Back 9

Holes	Par	Drive	Fairway	Putts	Hazard	Yardage	Strokes
10							
11							
12							
13							
14							
15							
16							
17							
18							
Total							
Grand Total							

Albatross	Eagles	Birdies	Pars	Bogeys	Doubles	Triples

Notes

Date _________________ Start time _________ End time _______

Course Name		
Weather	Temp	
Handicap	Par	
Tees	Yardage	
Players		

Front 9

Holes	Par	Drive	Fairway	Putts	Hazard	Yardage	Strokes
1							
2							
3							
4							
5							
6							
7							
8							
9							
Total							

Back 9

Holes	Par	Drive	Fairway	Putts	Hazard	Yardage	Strokes
10							
11							
12							
13							
14							
15							
16							
17							
18							
Total							
Grand Total							

Albatross	Eagles	Birdies	Pars	Bogeys	Doubles	Triples

Notes

Date _______________ Start time _________ End time _________

Course Name	
Weather	Temp
Handicap	Par
Tees	Yardage
Players	

Front 9							
Holes	Par	Drive	Fairway	Putts	Hazard	Yardage	Strokes
1							
2							
3							
4							
5							
6							
7							
8							
9							
Total							
Back 9							
10							
11							
12							
13							
14							
15							
16							
17							
18							
Total							
Grand Total							

Albatross	Eagles	Birdies	Pars	Bogeys	Doubles	Triples

Notes

Date _______________ Start time _________ End time _________

Course Name

Weather | Temp

Handicap | Par

Tees | Yardage

Players

Front 9							
Holes	Par	Drive	Fairway	Putts	Hazard	Yardage	Strokes
1							
2							
3							
4							
5							
6							
7							
8							
9							
Total							
Back 9							
10							
11							
12							
13							
14							
15							
16							
17							
18							
Total							
Grand Total							

Albatross	Eagles	Birdies	Pars	Bogeys	Doubles	Triples

Notes

Date _________________ Start time _________ End time _________

Course Name	
Weather	Temp
Handicap	Par
Tees	Yardage
Players	

Front 9

Holes	Par	Drive	Fairway	Putts	Hazard	Yardage	Strokes
1							
2							
3							
4							
5							
6							
7							
8							
9							
Total							

Back 9

Holes	Par	Drive	Fairway	Putts	Hazard	Yardage	Strokes
10							
11							
12							
13							
14							
15							
16							
17							
18							
Total							
Grand Total							

Albatross	Eagles	Birdies	Pars	Bogeys	Doubles	Triples

Notes

Course Name	
Weather	Temp
Handicap	Par
Tees	Yardage
Players	

Front 9

Holes	Par	Drive	Fairway	Putts	Hazard	Yardage	Strokes
1							
2							
3							
4							
5							
6							
7							
8							
9							
Total							

Back 9

Holes	Par	Drive	Fairway	Putts	Hazard	Yardage	Strokes
10							
11							
12							
13							
14							
15							
16							
17							
18							
Total							
Grand Total							

	Albatross	Eagles	Birdies	Pars	Bogeys	Doubles	Triples

Notes

Date _________________ Start time _________ End time _________

Course Name

Weather   Temp

Handicap   Par

Tees   Yardage

Players

Front 9

Holes	Par	Drive	Fairway	Putts	Hazard	Yardage	Strokes
1							
2							
3							
4							
5							
6							
7							
8							
9							
Total							

Back 9

Holes	Par	Drive	Fairway	Putts	Hazard	Yardage	Strokes
10							
11							
12							
13							
14							
15							
16							
17							
18							
Total							
Grand Total							

	Albatross	Eagles	Birdies	Pars	Bogeys	Doubles	Triples

Notes

Date _________________ Start time _________ End time _________

Course Name	
Weather	Temp
Handicap	Par
Tees	Yardage
Players	

Front 9

Holes	Par	Drive	Fairway	Putts	Hazard	Yardage	Strokes
1							
2							
3							
4							
5							
6							
7							
8							
9							
Total							

Back 9

Holes	Par	Drive	Fairway	Putts	Hazard	Yardage	Strokes
10							
11							
12							
13							
14							
15							
16							
17							
18							
Total							
Grand Total							

Albatross	Eagles	Birdies	Pars	Bogeys	Doubles	Triples

Notes

www.ingramcontent.com/pod-product-compliance
Lightning Source LLC
Chambersburg PA
CBHW031257250726
48655CB00005B/2258